All About
FEEDING OLDER PEOPLE

By Laura Flynn R.N., B.N., M.B.A., in consultation with her nurse educator associates and physicians who assisted in contributing and editing.

ISBN No: 978 1 896616 69 8

© 2011, 2017 Mediscript Communications Inc.

The publisher, Mediscript Communications Inc., acknowledges the financial support of the Government of Canada through the Canadian Book Fund for our publishing activities.

www.mediscript.net

Printed in Canada

Book and Front Cover design by:
Brian Adamson, www.AdamsonGraphics.net

7

FOP202011

ALL ABOUT BOOKS
Trusted • Reliable • Certified

- 40+ titles available
- Comply with accreditation and regulatory bodies
- Suitable for caregivers, boomers with elderly parents, health workers, auxiliary health staff & patients
- Self study style with "test yourself" section
- Health On the Net (HON) certified
- A person or patient seeking information on nutrition and self care.

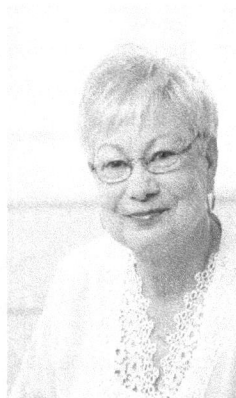

Some of our titles:

Alzheimers Disease	Arthritis	Multiple Sclerosis
Pain	Strokes	Elder Abuse
Falls Prevention	Incontinence	Nutrition & Aging
Personal Care	Positioning	Confusion
Transferring People	Care of the Back	Skin Care

For complete list of titles go to www.mediscript.net

Contact: 1 800 773 5088
Fax 1800 639 3186 • Email: mediscript30@yahoo.ca

CONTENTS

INTRODUCTION

This book provides basic, non controversial and trusted information that can help a wide spectrum of readers.

The primary objective of the information is to help a person provide effective quality care to a loved one or someone in his or her care.

Your role as a caregiver could mean the older person in your care is a family member or loved one, or you may be a non family member who is helping out a friend. Alternatively, you may be a paid health worker providing quality care for a client. With this in mind, we will alternate between referring to family members, loved ones, older persons and clients.

All the information is reliable and was written by a group of eminent nurse educators who ensured the information complies with best practice guidelines and satisfies the various accreditation and regulatory bodies. Because there is so much unreliable information on the internet, you can be assured the "All About" publications are HON (Health On the Net) certified.

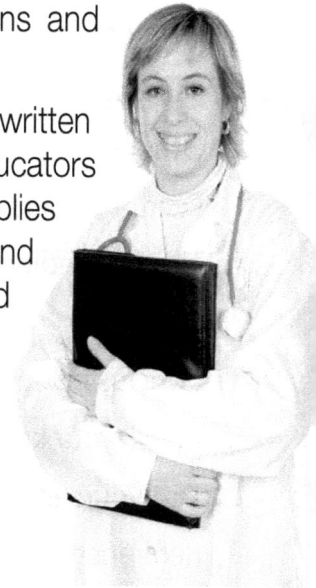

AN IMPORTANT MESSAGE FROM THE PUBLISHER

Each person's treatment, advice, medical aids, physical therapy and other approaches to health care are unique and highly dependant upon the diagnosis and overall assessment by the medical team.

We emphasize therefore that the information within this book is not a substitute for the advice and treatment from a health care professional.

After reading this material you will have a better understanding of the common feeding problems of older people. As well, you will be more prepared to assist the people in your care to a better quality of life.

With all this in mind, the publishers and authors disclaim any responsibility for any adverse effects resulting directly or indirectly from the suggestions contained within this book or from any misunderstanding of the content on the part of the reader.

Actual Medical Records

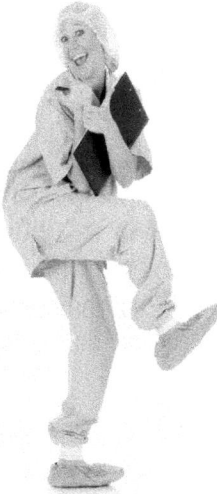

- Healthy appearing decrepit 69 year-old male, mentally alert but forgetful.

- She slipped on the ice and apparently her legs went in separate directions in early December.

- The patient had waffles for breakfast and anorexia for lunch.

- Patient was seen in consultation by Dr. Jones, who felt that we should sit on the abdomen and I agree.

HOW MUCH DO YOU KNOW?

It helps to figure out how much you know before you start. In this way you will have an idea as to the gaps in your knowledge prior to reading the content. Please circle to indicate the best answer. Remember, at this stage, you are not expected to know all the answers:

1. Dysphagia means having a poor appetite.

a) True

b) False

2. Which of the following promotes the social aspect of eating?

a) Sitting next to the person while eating.

b) Allowing the person to watch TV while eating.

c) Standing over the person while feeding him/her.

d) Setting the pace of the meal for the person.

3. Tea is a good choice for people who have difficulty swallowing.

a) True

b) False

4. Mixing food together in a blender will improve the taste.

a) True

b) False

5. Mr. Taylor has difficulty swallowing. Which of the following strategies is appropriate?

a) Sit him upright during the meal.

b) Allow him to lie down when he's finished eating.

c) Use a straw to give him fluids.

d) A and C

6. A decreased sense of smell can interfere with appetite.

a) True

b) False

7. Small frequent meals are better than large meals if the person has a poor appetite.

a) True

b) False

ANSWERS

1. b. False. Dysphagia means difficulty swallowing.

2. a. Eating is a social activity and people may have to eat alone in their rooms. Sitting next to the person helps to make it feel like more of a social experience.

3. b. False. Thin liquids, like tea and water, can splash against the back of the throat before the person is ready to swallow.

4. b. False. Serve one food at a time rather than mixing different foods.

5. a. Sitting in an upright position when he eats or drink will help to prevent choking and allow gravity to assist the food moving into his stomach.

6. a. True. The smell of food plays a large part in our enjoyment of eating.

7. a. True. Provide small frequent meals if the person has a poor appetite.

SOMETHING TO THINK ABOUT...

When I am employed in servingothers,

I do not look upon myself as conferring

favors but paying debts.

Benjamin Franklin

FEEDING OLDER PEOPLE

Have you ever heard the saying "You are what you eat"? There is a great deal of truth in that statement. The foods that we eat on a daily basis have a great impact on our state of health. Nutrition is very important for good health.

Eating healthy foods helps people to recover from illness or surgery, to maintain their present state of health or to achieve a higher level of health status. Good nutrition involves more than just serving healthy meals, however. Elderly people often cannot, or do not, eat the foods they are given.

People who are away from familiar surroundings may have poor appetites. They may have illnesses or be on medications that decrease their appetites. The hospital or long-term care agencies may have unusual sights and smells. Food can be different. People lose control over food choices and how food is prepared. People in long term care residences are expected to eat when meals are served and the timing of the meal may not be what they're used to. For many people, eating is a social activity and people may have to eat alone in their rooms. All of these factors can affect a person's eating patterns.

Whether they're living at home or in a long term care residence, older people frequently require assistance with their meals. They may be unable to feed themselves because of overall weakness, paralysis, or confusion. Or they may be able to feed themselves, but will need help preparing their meal trays. You can have a major impact on an older person's nutrition by knowing how to provide assistance and encouragement at mealtime.

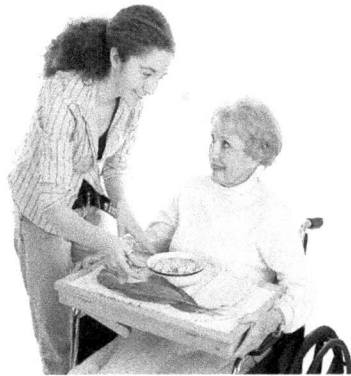

CONSIDER FOR A MOMENT ...

Have you had problems in the past

when assisting older people

at mealtimes?

What types of problems have you had?

HELPING SOMEONE WITH A POOR APPETITE

Outlined in the next few chapters are several examples of feeding problems that caregivers often come across. Each case example has follow-up questions. Try to answer the questions on your own before reading the discussion following each example.

CASE EXAMPLE

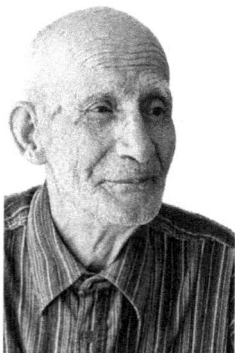

Mr. Angel is 76 years old. He lives at home. He has breathing and heart problems and requires some help with daily activities. You provide care to him in his home. Mr. Angel has a poor appetite. You prepare his meals, but he is able to feed himself.

CONSIDER FOR A MOMENT ...

Take a few minutes to consider what you could do to help someone like Mr. Angel improve his appetite. Then read the following discussion.

Many things can cause a poor appetite. Mr. Angel may be on many medications that can interfere with his appetite. Because of his medical condition, he may not be very active. Mr. Angel may have decreased taste and smell as a normal change of aging. He may be depressed or lonely. His dentures may not fit properly. He may be tired.

Monitor Mr. Angel's food intake and eating habits. Note what foods he likes and dislikes. Ask him if he can smell and taste his food. Provide small, frequent meals. Ask him what times he would like his meals. Find out when he is hungriest and give him the largest meal at that time. Throughout the day, encourage Mr. Angel to have as much activity as possible. This may help to make him hungry.

Try to make his meals look and smell as nice as possible. Remove any clutter from the table and set it properly. Arrange the food so he can easily reach it. Ensure he has his glasses and dentures. Make sure there is good lighting so he can see his food. Provide encouragement for him to eat. "Maybe you could try to eat just half of the sandwich for now."

Make sure he is comfortable during the meal. He should be seated comfortably. If possible, try to schedule medications so that they do not interfere with his meals. Medications that taste bad or those that may make him feel sick should not be given just before meals. (You may have to discuss this with your supervisor or Mr. Angel's healthcare professional.) Encourage him to brush his teeth and to wash his face and hands before the meal. Brushing his teeth will improve his ability to taste the food. Washing his face and hands may make him feel better.

Make his meals as enjoyable as possible. Make sure there are no unpleasant sights or smells while he is eating. If he enjoys company, sit with him. Talk to him about pleasant topics. If he likes music, play whatever he enjoys.

If you are caring for someone like Mr. Angel in an institution, use similar strategies. It might be more difficult to provide small, frequent meals with food that your client likes in an institution. However, you must still try. Tell the dietitian everything you know about your client's eating habits. Encourage the family to bring in home cooked meals that the client likes whenever possible.

When you are caring for someone who is not interested in eating, try to find out why. Not feeling well? Don't like the food? Eaten recently – maybe the family brought in a snack? For people who refuse to eat or who constantly spit food out, provide a drink. Return later, about 10-20 minutes, and try again. Provide nourishing snacks and drinks between meals.

Many people at home or in institutions are lonely and eat much better when in the company of friends or family. If you are caring for someone who seems lonely, encourage him/her to call family or friends and invite them to visit and share a meal.

HELPING SOMEONE WHO CAN SELF-FEED

CASE EXAMPLE

Mrs. Johnson is confined to bed in a long-term care facility. She is weak, but can feed herself with some assistance setting up her tray.

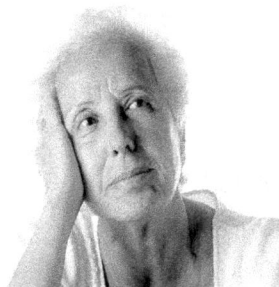

CONSIDER FOR A MOMENT ...

Consider what steps you could follow to assist Mrs. Johnson. Then read the discussion on the next page.

Try to arrange rest periods before meals if Mrs. Johnson appears tired at mealtimes. Ensure that she is as comfortable as possible. For anyone who experiences pain, contact a healthcare professional regarding pain medications.

Before giving the tray to Mrs. Johnson, ask her if she has any special habits she likes to do before she eats. Offer the bedpan to her. Help her to wash her face and hands. Assist Mrs. Johnson into a sitting position. This will make her feel more comfortable and will help her see and access her meal. Also, it will be more difficult for her to open her mouth, chew, and swallow if she is slumped over.

Elevate the head of the bed or support Mrs. Johnson with pillows. Position the overbed table across the bed so she can easily access her meal. (Tip: If Mrs. Johnson were in her own home and did not have an overbed table, an ironing board could be used!) Ensure she is wearing her dentures and glasses. Offer oral care by helping her to brush her teeth or use mouthwash.

Wash your hands before you touch Mrs. Johnson's tray. Check the name on the tray to make sure that the tray is the one Mrs. Johnson is supposed to have. Place the tray so Mrs. Johnson can reach it easily.

Prepare her tray by opening milk or juice cartons and by removing lids. If she needs extra help, cut her meat, butter the bread, and prepare hot fluids (tea, coffee) for her.

Allow Mrs. Johnson to do as much as possible for herself. Being able to feed oneself promotes independence and self-worth. Remember that Mrs. Johnson is an adult. Treat her with dignity. Avoid scolding her, or any other client, for poor eating habits.

Following the meal, note what was eaten and how much. Assist Mrs. Johnson to wash her face and hands. Also assist with oral hygiene. Ensure that she is comfortable and that her call bell is within easy reach.

HELPING SOMEONE WHO IS CONFUSED

CASE EXAMPLE

Harold Digby is 74 years old. He lives at home and has 24-hour home care. Mr. Digby is becoming more and more confused. He is physically able to feed himself, but sometimes it seems he does not remember how.

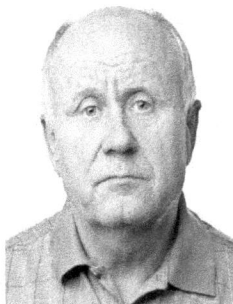

CONSIDER FOR A MOMENT ...

Consider what steps you could take to assist Mr. Digby. Then compare your ideas with the ones begining on the next page.

Establish a routine and follow it at all mealtimes. Mr. Digby should eat his meals at the same time and in the same place. If he usually has his meals in the dining room, he should always have his meals there. Keep necessary items, such as a napkin and utensils, in the same place for each meal. Mr. Digby should sit in the same place for all of his meals.

Avoid distractions at mealtimes. Noise may distract him from eating. Turn off the television and ensure there are no loud noises. Patterns may also be distracting so use plain tablecloths, napkins, placemats, and dishes.

Provide lots of encouragement during the meal. Give him simple instructions. "Take a bite of chicken. O.K., now swallow." Mr. Digby may forget how to use the utensils for meals. Make sure he knows how to use the fork and spoon.

Offer only one plate and one utensil at a time rather than the complete tray. This reduces the decisions and choices Mr. Digby has to make about what and how to eat. Finger foods are easier for him to eat. A bowl will be easier than a plate (he may push food off the plate as he tries to get it on the fork). Fill cups so they are only half full. This will help to reduce the number of spills.

As with all confused clients, ensure Mr. Digby's safety during the meal. Ensure the food and fluids are not too hot. Prepare hot drinks for him so he will not be burned. Cut his food into small bites. Stay close as he is eating to ensure he does not have any problems with choking.

FEEDING A DEPENDENT PERSON

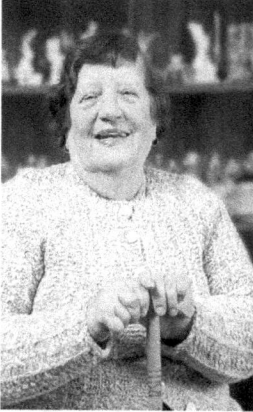

CASE EXAMPLE

Mrs. Ryan has an illness that causes severe weakness in her muscles. She has been in the long-term care agency for about 4 months. She is aware of her surroundings and can speak. She cannot feed herself.

CONSIDER FOR A MOMENT ...

Consider what you could do to make mealtime more enjoyable for someone who cannot feed herself and cannot speak. How would you like to be treated if you were in Mrs. Ryan's situation? Compare your thoughts with the ones on the following pages.

Before feeding anyone, always check the care plan. Does the person have any food allergies? Any special diet? Any special eating habits? Wash your hands before touching the tray.

Having to be fed can be a blow to a person's self-esteem. It can cause a person to feel helpless. Mrs. Ryan may have feelings of loss of control. It is important to treat her with dignity. Treat older people who are being fed as adults, not as children.

Use a napkin, not a bib to cover her clothes. If a bib must be used, make sure it is not childish looking. Serve foods prepared as normally as possible. Only blend food if Mrs. Ryan's condition requires it this way. Using bibs and blending foods together decrease a person's dignity. Ensure she has her glasses on so she can see the food. Involve her in the feeding process as much as possible. Allow her to hold the straw, if she can, while you hold the cup for her.

While feeding Mrs. Ryan, ask what she would like to eat next. "Would you like potatoes or peas now?"

Allow her to direct the pace of the meal. Let her know if the food is hot or cold. Offer fluids after every three or four mouthfuls of food. Ensure food and liquids are at the right temperature. If it is supposed to be hot, make sure it is hot, but not too hot. Continue to check the temperature of the food throughout the meal.

Try to make the surroundings as pleasant as possible. If Mrs. Ryan likes to hear music during meals, ask her what she would like to hear and turn it on for her. Talk to her about pleasant topics during the meal.

Feeding someone, or assisting someone to eat, can be very time-consuming. However, make sure Mrs. Ryan does not think that you are in a rush. She should not feel that it is a bother for you to have to feed her. Sit opposite Mrs. Ryan, instead of standing over her. Don't put too much food on the fork. Piling food onto the fork can lead to food spills and difficulties with chewing or swallowing. Offer fluids regularly. Allow Mrs. Ryan enough time to chew the food and swallow before offering the next forkful.

Following the meal, help Mrs. Ryan wash her face and hands and brush her teeth. Position her comfortably. Ensure her call bell is within easy reach.

Sometimes people have medical conditions that make it necessary for them to stay in bed while being fed. They may not be able to fully sit up while in bed. When that happens, slow and careful feeding is even more important to prevent choking.

If you work in a health care facility, have you ever been in a situation where many clients needed help with their meals but only a few staff were available to assist? This type of situation can affect clients' nutrition. Some of the results that have been observed include:

• Clients were fed more often in bed to save time;

• Clients were not always positioned properly;

• The meal tray was poorly positioned;

• Food got cold;

• Very little talking took place during mealtime;

• Clients were not carefully cleaned before and after meals;

• Clients were not fed as much as they should have been;

• Clients were fed too quickly with too much on the fork;

• All of the food was mixed together so it could be eaten more quickly;

- Clients found mealtimes frightening rather than pleasant;

- Clients were not given enough time to feed themselves; and

- Clients were not encouraged to eat.

It may be possible to have volunteers or family members assist with feeding. Check the institution's policy regarding this. Make sure whoever is feeding the person is aware of the client's eating rituals or special eating needs. Talk with your supervisor if you think you have too many people too feed at one time.

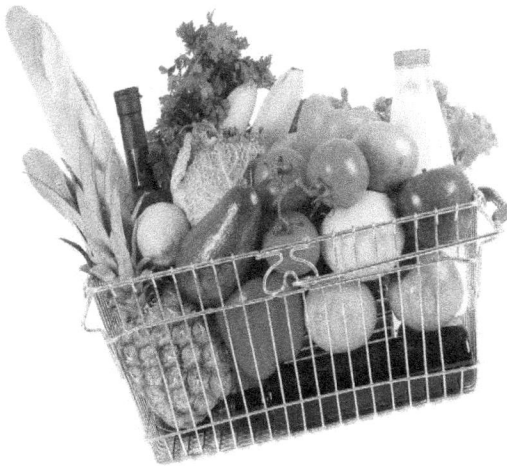

OTHER PROBLEMS

Dentures that don't fit well

A lack of teeth or dentures that don't fit well can make chewing difficult. Red gums may be a sign that dentures are not fitting properly. Chop foods finely to reduce chewing. Offer softer foods. Select foods carefully; for example ground meat or fish is easier to chew than steak. Talk with the supervisor regarding getting dentures that fit properly.

Decreased sense of taste and smell

Provide mouth care before the meal. Serve one food at a time rather than mixing different foods. Serve foods with different textures. Foods with strong flavours and aromas may help. Add sweeteners or herbs to boost the flavour.

People who are blind

Tell the person where the food is located on the plate by comparing the location to a clock. For example, the chicken is at 12:00, the carrots are at 3:00, the potatoes are at 7:00.

People who need help with utensils

Use normal eating utensils whenever possible. However, pain, stiffness, or deformed joints can decrease ability to grip cups or utensils. Lack of muscle control, weakness, paralysis, or a tremor (or shake) can also cause a decreased grip. Pain or stiffness in arms can make it difficult to bring a cup to one's mouth. Stiffness in the neck can make it painful to tip one's head forward to eat or drink.

Use special utensils if it gives the person more independence. If you are involved in helping to select special eating equipment, make sure it is practical. Is it easy to clean? Can it be washed in the dishwasher? Can it be used in the microwave? How sturdy is it? Will it break if it falls or is tipped over?

Forks, spoons, and knives with wide handles are easier to grip. Hand straps also work if the grip is weak. It is easier to keep food in a deep spoon. It is also possible to get utensils that combine the fork, spoon, and knife into one tool. A pizza cutter can be easier to use than a knife to cut food. Use finger foods that don't require utensils whenever possible.

Cups with large handles or those with two handles are easier to hold. Cups that are only partly filled are easier to manage. Drinking cups that have spouts or others that have lids with small holes help to reduce spills. Straws can also make it easier for the person to drink. A terrycloth wristband over a glass or cup makes it easier to hold. Ribbed glasses are also easier to hold. Sturdy cups or glasses will not be as easy to tip over.

Plates with rims, or a bowl, allow food to be pushed against them so it is easier to get the food on the fork or spoon. Suction on the bottom of plates or bowls helps to keep them in place. A damp cloth under the plate also works.

CONSIDER FOR A MOMENT ...

Have you ever cared for people with other feeding problems that are not mentioned above?

DYSPHAGIA

What is dysphagia?

Dysphagia means difficulty swallowing. It occurs more often in the elderly. 40-60% of older adults in institutions have signs of dysphagia. Such clients have been called "difficult" or "uncooperative" because they were not eating quickly.

Dysphagia can cause food to leak or spill out of the mouth. It can lead to poor nutrition and weight loss. People can get pneumonia if food goes into the lungs. Feelings of shame are possible and a person with dysphagia may not want to eat with other people around.

Dysphagia can be caused by confusion. Some illnesses, such as strokes, that can lead to weakness and paralysis of the face can also cause it. Some medications can cause it. Having many teeth missing and no dentures or poorly fitting dentures can also lead to dysphagia.

What are the signs of dysphagia?

The signs of dysphagia include:

• needing to swallow several times after each bite;

• coughing or choking before, during, or after swallowing;

• complaining of having something stuck in the throat;

• constant drooling;

• food leaking from the mouth;

• food being kept in the mouth;

• drooping face;

• difficulty closing lips;

• having a hoarse or gurgling voice, and

• resisting being fed.

How can you help a client with dysphagia?

You are caring for Mrs. Lee. She had a stroke several months ago. Mrs. Lee has a lot of difficulty swallowing. She requires assistance when she eats or drinks.

What can you do to help Mrs. Lee during meals?

There are several strategies. To begin, she should be supervised when she eats. She should be sitting in an upright position when she eats or drinks. This helps to prevent choking and allows gravity to assist the food moving into her stomach. Only feed her when she is wide awake. She should wear well-fitting dentures.

She should chew her food thoroughly. Offer only small bites of food. Food should be placed on the unaffected side of her face. Give her plenty of time to eat. Provide brief instructions to remind Mrs. Lee to chew and swallow. She may need a reminder to close her teeth and lips before trying to swallow. If necessary, help close her mouth with your hand.

If Mrs. Lee also has difficulty chewing, serve soft foods. Put food through a blender or food processor, but only if necessary. Food that requires gentle swallowing may be better than food that has been pureed (blended). It may trigger movement of the tongue and mouth, which can help swallowing. As well, food that is not pureed is usually more acceptable.

Serve thick liquids. Thick liquids are easier to swallow. Thin liquids, such as water and tea, should be avoided. Thin liquids can splash against the back of the throat before the person is ready to swallow. Don't use straws. Dry foods such as crackers should be avoided. Sticky foods such as peanut butter should be avoided.

Some people will need to concentrate when trying to swallow. Provide pleasant surroundings that are free from distractions. Keep conversation to a minimum if needed. Mrs. Lee should not talk when trying to swallow. Avoid asking her questions during the meal. It may be better to feed her in her room if the dining room is noisy.

Following the meal, check Mrs. Lee's mouth to ensure all food has been swallowed. Provide mouth care following the meal. Keep her sitting up for at least 30-60 minutes to prevent food from going into the lungs.

Talk to your supervisor or health care professional if you are having difficulty feeding someone or if you have concerns about someone's ability to swallow.

Remember that every person is an individual. Depending upon the cause of the dysphagia and how serious the person's condition is, certain foods may or may not be appropriate.

Some of the techniques mentioned here may not be used in every situation. The health professional can assist to develop an appropriate feeding plan for you to follow.

CONSIDER FOR A MOMENT ...

Have you ever cared for someone with dysphagia? Are you caring for someone now whom you think may have dysphagia?

TIPS FOR FEEDING CLIENTS
WITH DYSPHAGIA

The following are general tips that may help when feeding older people with dysphagia:

- Supervise during mealtime.

- Sit the person upright.

- Only feed when he or she is wide awake.

- Ensure dentures fit well.

- Encourage the person to chew food well.

- Offer only small bites of food.

- Place food on the unaffected side of the face.

- Allow the person plenty of time to eat.

- Remind the person to chew and swallow.

- Serve soft foods if he or she has difficulty chewing.

- Serve thick liquids. Thick liquids are easier to swallow. Thin liquids, such as water and tea, should be avoided.

- Don't use straws.

- Avoid dry foods such as crackers.

- Provide pleasant surroundings that are free from distractions.

- Avoid asking questions during the meal. People with swallowing difficulties need to concentrate at mealtime.

- Check the person's mouth after meals to ensure all food has been swallowed.

- Provide mouth care after the meal.

- Keep the person sitting up for at least 30-60 minutes after the meal to prevent food from going into the lungs.

- Let your supervisor or health care professional know if you notice that anyone in your care is having swallowing problems. A health care professional should assess the person.

Remember that every person is an individual. Some of the tips mentioned above may not be suitable depending upon the cause of the dysphagia and how serious the person's condition is. As well, you may have to follow guidelines that are not mentioned above for other people. Follow the care plan and doctor's orders for the person in your care.

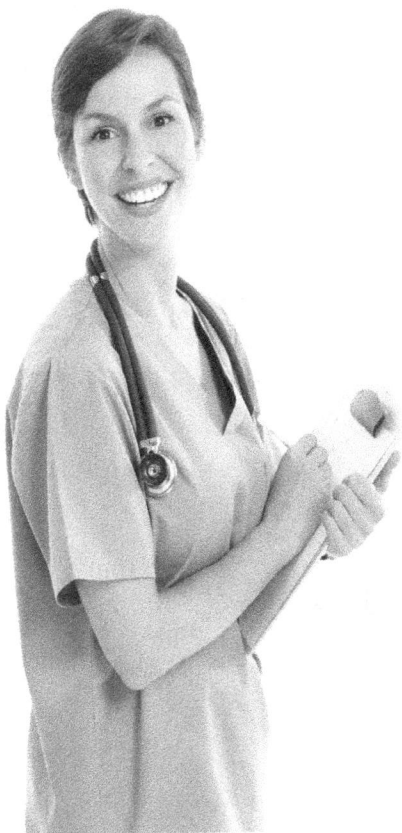

CONCLUSION

Dining is often thought of as a social event. Self-feeding should be encouraged as long as possible. When assisting someone to eat, only do what absolutely has to be done. If the person can feed him/herself with only verbal encouragement, then just provide that. If he or she only needs help with taking the lids off containers or cutting meat, do so.

Try to make the meal as normal as possible. Have pleasant surroundings, such as gentle music. Try to arrange for the person to eat in the dining room instead of the bedroom. Assist him into a chair rather than eating in bed. Use standard utensils and dishes if possible. Use napkins rather than bibs. Allow him to be as involved as possible. Provide help and assistance thoughtfully.

Try to be discreet about feeding if the person has company. Allow the person in your care as much control as possible over the meal. Sit next to her and allow her to set the pace of the meal and to make choices about what to eat next and when to drink.

Be alert to any difficulties he or she may be having while eating. Note what is eaten and how much. By providing thoughtful assistance and encouragement at mealtime, you can have a major effect on the nutrition of the person you are caring for.

SOMETHING TO THINK ABOUT...

A man's true wealth is the good he does in this world.

Mohammed

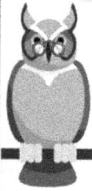

CHECK YOUR KNOWLEDGE

1. What strategies can you use to improve a person's appetite?

2. What steps should you take to help someone who is bedridden but can feed himself?

3. What 4 strategies can you use to promote someone's independence during eating?

4. What utensils would help a person who has a decreased grip?

5. What strategies can you use to assist a confused person to feed herself?

6. What is dysphagia?

7. How should you feed a person who has difficulty swallowing?

TEST YOURSELF

Please circle to indicate the best answer:

1. Difficulty swallowing is a common problem of elderly clients in institutions.

a) True

b) False

2. Which of the following can cause a poor appetite in an elderly person?

a) Illnesses

b) Medications

c) Decreased activity

d) All of the above

3. A person has had a stroke and has a droop on one side of her face. Food should be placed on the affected side of her face.

a) True

b) False

4. Which of the following will help someone with decreased taste?

a) Use sweeteners and herbs to promote flavor

b) Provide mouth care before meals

c) Serve food with strong flavors

d) A and C

e) All of the above

5. Which of the following should help the person while she is being fed?

a) Allow the person to choose what she eats next

b) Give her plenty of time

c) Let her lie down on her side as she is being fed

d) A and B

e) All of the above

6. Comparing the location of a blind person's food to a clock will help the person to eat.

a) True

b) False

7. Distractions during eating should be limited for the confused person.

a) True

b) False

ANSWERS

1. a. True. 40-60% of older adults in institutions have signs of dysphagia.

2. d. Illnesses, medications, and decreased activity are all factors that can contribute to a loss of appetite.

3. b. False. Food should be placed on the unaffected side of her face.

4. e. These are all aids to improving the flavour of food and encouraging the person to eat.

5. d. Give the person plenty of time and allow her to choose what she eats next.

6. a. True. For example, tell the person the chicken is at 12:00, the carrots are at 3:00, the potatoes are at 7:00.

7. a. True. Noise, such as the TV, may distract him from eating. Patterns may also be distracting so use plain tablecloths, napkins, placemats, and dishes.

REFERENCES

Amella, E. J. (1998). Assessment and management of eating and feeding difficulties for older people: A NICHE protocol. Geriatric Nursing, 19(5), 269-275.

Caregiver Education and Support Services. (1990). Caregiver's handbook (Part 4). Retrieved January 29, 2002 from http://www.acsu.buffalo.edu/~drstall/hndbk4.html

Craven, R.F., & Hirnle, C. J. (2000). Fundamentals of nursing: Human health and function (3rd ed., pp. 717-718, 943-944). Philadelphia, PA: Lippincott.

Disabled Living Foundation. (1998). Choosing eating and drinking equipment. Retrieved January 29, 2002 from http://factsheets.disabledliving.org.uk/choosing-eating-and-drinking-equipment/

Jacobsson, C., Axelsson, K., Norberg, A., Asplund, K., & Wenngren, B. (1997). Outcomes of individualized interventions in patients with severe eating difficulties. Clinical Nursing Research, 6(1), 25-44.

Kayser-Jones, J., & Schell, E. (1997). The effect of staffing on the quality of care at mealtime. Nursing Outlook, 45(2), 64-72.

Kayser-Jones, J., & Pengilly, K. (1999). Dysphagia among nursing home clients. Geriatric Nursing, 20(2), 77-82.

Kozier, B., Erb, G., Berman, A., & Burke, K. (2000). Fundamentals of nursing: Concepts, process, and practice (6th ed., pp. 1146-1148). Upper Saddle River, NJ: Prentice Hall Health.

Maas, M.L., Buckwalter, K.C., Hardy, M.D., Tripp-Reimer, T., Titler, M.G., & Specht, J.P. (2001). Nursing care of older adults: Diagnoses, outcomes, & interventions. St. Louis, Missouri: Mosby.

Meyer, M., & Derr, P. (1998). The comfort of home: An illustrated step-by-step guide for caregivers (pp. 192-196). Portland, Oregon: CareTrust Publications.

Miller, C.A. (1999). Nursing care of older adults – Theory & practice (3rd ed.). Philadelphia, PA: Lippincott.

Senior Care Web. (2000). Responsibilities: Assisting with eating. Retrieved January 29, 2002 from http://www2.seniorcareweb.com/senior/caregiverissue/responsibiliti/cgeating.htm

Taylor, C., Lillis, C., & LeMone, P. (2001). Fundamentals of nursing: The art & science of nursing care (4th ed., pp. 1104-1106). Philadelphia, PA: Lippincott.

www.ingramcontent.com/pod-product-compliance
Lightning Source LLC
Chambersburg PA
CBHW071757200326
41520CB00013BA/3286